Gorgeous SKIN

Gorgeous SKIN

What You Need to Know to Have Beautiful Skin Every Day

Dr. Sonya Campbell Johnson

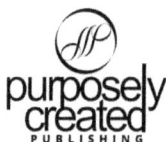

purposely
created
PUBLISHING

GORGEOUS SKIN
Published by Purposely Created Publishing Group™
Copyright © 2020 Sonya Campbell Johnson

All rights reserved.

Unless otherwise indicated, scripture quotations are from the Holy Bible, King James Version. All rights reserved.

Printed in the United States of America
ISBN: 978-1-64484-196-9

Special discounts are available on bulk quantity purchases by book clubs, associations and special interest groups. For details email: sales@publishyourgift.com or call (888) 949-6228. *For information log on to:* www.PublishYourGift.com

This book is dedicated to my parents, Mary Ann and Jesse Louis Campbell, who told me I could do all things through God who strengthens me (Philippians 4:13 KJV). My sister, Felicia Pleshette, who reassures me I'm more than enough. My deceased sister, Jessica Anastasia Louise, whose memory encourages me to live and enjoy all that God has in this world for us and to engage in life. My sons, LJ and Sharif, who always tell me I am beautiful and a great mom. While ushering them into manhood, I blossomed.

Table of Contents

Introduction

My intention for this book is to empower women of color who have skin problems by sharing my knowledge about the skin. The information contained here will help them know what it takes to clear their skin and develop even skin tone for life. I want them to experience what it feels like to be stress free and choose to go bare skinned in public. My desire is for them to experience the freedom of wearing make-up as an option, not as a necessity.

I graduated top of my high school class, served as one of the medical school admissions committee members, was co-chief resident for dermatology, and started my practice one year after graduating from dermatology residency. I have been in private practice for 20 years and have three locations. I have performed numerous surgeries and other procedures.

Can I become vulnerable with you? As a single practitioner, problems arose when the government started making demands on physicians, and employee turnover and overhead cost increased, while reimbursements from insurance companies decreased. Have you ever felt exhausted from your job? Lost the desire to go to work? Have you ever felt alone, bitter, or resentful? Have you ever experienced a lack of security? I started having medical problems such as insomnia, weight gain, and development of digestive problems. After lying in bed with severe abdominal pain, I realized something had to change. After acknowledging all of my new medical problems, I decided to get a grip on my life and situation. I considered selling my practice in hopes of feeling more secure. I narrowed the scope and went on a tour of a potential buyer. Days later, while walking in the park, my lawyer called.

It was one of those heart-to-heart, authentic conversations. I do not remember asking for her opinion, but she gave it, nevertheless. She told me I was looking for security, and I was not going to find it at any large medical group and definitely not any hospital. After analyzing all the information presented to me, I realized she was correct. Hospitals purchase practices, but I saw firsthand how they fired physicians or physicians left because they were not appreciated. The large dermatology groups also fired physicians after acquiring their practices, or the physician would quit from being overworked. With both options, the physician lost all autonomy. I remember asking God, "What is it that you wanted me to see while visiting other practices?" What I saw and put into practice changed my world. I changed my mindset, acquired new skills, changed my office paradigm, hired a business coach, and started engaging in social media. I started really listening to my patients, and all of them wanted clear skin and even skin tone with increased confidence. From there, I created products and performed procedures that resulted in clear and even skin tones for my clients. I realized I wanted to share my gifts with the world. Within months everything started changing for my office.

Now, I am a highly sought-after dermatologist and national speaker who helps women of color who have concerns with their complexion, performs Mohs Micrographic surgery, and treats any skin problem for all ages and ethnic groups.

Chapter 1

BEAUTY MINDSET

Beauty: is it in the eye of the beholder? What is your definition of beauty? Is it the outward appearance of a person or the inward appearance that is personified outwardly? Everyone has their own meaning when they define beauty. That is why it is so important for you to define beauty on your own terms and exemplify what beauty is for you. Once you have your own definition of beauty and demonstrate it in your everyday life, no one can make you what you do not want to be . . . only you can. Then and only then, can you change the areas of your skin you feel are problematic into something more appealing to you.

Our level of self-confidence is affected by many factors, our outward appearance, our work, our successes, or a supportive environment, to name a few. Since our society has placed an enormous value on our appearance, we are always determined to present ourselves in an acceptable fashion.

Self-confidence is shaped and developed at an early age. When girls are judged and comments are directed toward their appearance, skin, or beauty, they become more aware of the impact their beauty has on their environment and themselves. If society tells a girl she is not pretty, she believes it. It is only when we become self-aware, hear our own internal voice, and recognize our ability to change the negative connotation about ourselves, that we have the ability to disregard the negative voices. But when this does not happen, self-esteem and self-confidence are affected. We see this when adolescents develop acne or any visible skin problems. Young ladies feel inferior or unsure of themselves. Matters are worse if they are teased about their condition. The real problem is not the skin condition but how they view themselves and the aftermath of making poor decisions, followed by the development of low self-esteem to the point they miss out on life-changing opportunities because they did not exert themselves and instead became introverted or ashamed. Did their reaction to the skin condition or reaction to the negative comments create such a low self-image that it caused them to miss out on life's possibilities such as trying out for the cheerleading team or running for a school office? I have some clients who discuss how treating their severely acne-scarred skin changed their lives, not only the outward appearance but also internally through self-confidence. They felt more confident, alive, and excited about their potential. Beautiful skin, by their definition, helped them increase their self-confidence, giving them permission to do just about anything. From there, my clients shared how they became involved in activities they felt they would have otherwise disregarded because of their negative view of themselves and their disposition of being ashamed, if it was not for seeing a dermatologist who recommend products to clear their skin.

We talk about desires for our lives, our families, and our careers. But what about our skin? Have you really thought about this organ, the largest organ on your body, the one everyone can see? Yes, a large part of it is usually covered, but there is still enough skin exposed. Do you want to keep the skin marks to a minimal? Do you want to look younger than your real age? Do you even care? This is a simple but major question because it will help you keep things in perspective when you start to age and enter the land of trying to stay youthful in our judgmental society. To what degree are you willing to take care of yourself to avoid paying more in the future to keep your youthful appearance? Again, your definition of beauty and youthful appearance is your own definition and not what society has defined as beautiful and youthful. I have a client who wants to age gracefully, meaning she wants to look her best for her age not necessarily look younger. Once you are clear on your desires for your skin, you will know what actions to take whether that's monthly facials with a daily home regimen or ablative lasers because you started the process of taking care of your skin too late and now you need to play catch-up. Just remember, like any other goal we have for our lives, the skin is no different. It takes time to develop the changes you are working towards even if you have professional help. Professional services or procedures will shorten the length of time required to produce the desired outcomes for your skin, but it will still take time.

Even if you are basing the desired outcomes for your skin on your definition of beauty, you still need to be realistic about the outcomes and the duration it will take to reach your desired goals. If you spent several years baking in the sun to the point you have leathery skin, discoloration all over, or benign growths, do not expect the skin to return to pre-adolescent days. Some skin changes will never clear, but yes, you can achieve significant improvement but at a cost and unknown duration of time. If you have a wedding, do not wait until the week of the wedding to get procedures performed. It took time to develop the negative skin conditions, so it may take time to reverse the problem. We have to accept that aging is inevitable; however, we can slow the rate.

With so many options to choose from that can be used to change your outward appearance, you must keep a healthy thought process. Yes, you can have major procedures done to clear that acne bump on the cheek, but is it necessary or will a cream suffice? Unfortunately, doctors see clients who want major changes performed to their skin because they feel they are not attractive even though no apparent changes are needed. The problem is the clients do not know they have a dysmorphic view of themselves. Usually the sign of this disorder is visiting several doctors who see no concerns with one's skin. That's a clue. If you have a dysmorphic image of your body, it progresses to the point you have unnecessary procedures, leaving you at times worse off than before you started the process.

Chapter 2

SKIN DEVELOPMENT & MATURATION

The skin, the largest organ of the body, has several purposes. The skin is our first line of defense or a protective barrier. It protects us from toxins, pollutants, and radiation. The immune system in the skin fights harmful infestations. Our skin can identify and destroy foreign substances. Millions of pores in our skin have the ability to absorb oxygen, water, vitamins, and acids to provide moisture and nourishment to our bodies. The skin is the largest waste removal system. Through the pores and sweat glands, toxins are excreted. Sebum, secreted on the skin, is a mixture of oils that keep the skin soft and supple. Sebum or oil creates the acid mantle on the top layer of the skin. The acidic nature, with a pH of 4.5-5.5, protects the skin from outside invaders. The skin has regulatory functions in it that keep the body temperature at optimum levels. When the body's temperature increases, the skin produces water in the form of sweat, which evaporates releasing heat and cooling the body. When the body's temperature decreases, you notice goosebumps forming, shivering, and the muscles contract, giving off heat that warms the body. With nerve endings throughout the skin to transmit stimuli, our body stays in contact with the outside world through detecting sensations of cold, hot, pressure, and pain.

A single layer of cells that represent the evolving epidermis is seen as early as three weeks in the developing embryo. The skin is comprised of three layers: epidermis, dermis, and subcutaneous. Other structures present in the dermis and subcutaneous layer include the hair structure, nail unit, glands (apocrine-scent, eccrine-sweat, sebaceous-oil, lacrimal-tear, and mammary-milk glands), melanocytes, and Langerhans cells (fight infections). Sex hormones affecting the skin can be seen early with the development of the sebaceous glands. The sebaceous glands are well-formed in neonates by the effects of the maternal androgen that crosses the placenta barrier. It causes the sebaceous glands to develop and stimulate the cells to make lipids. This only occurs until the maternal androgen levels fall, which is within a couple of weeks. Then the sebaceous glands decrease in size considerably. As an infant, the external environmental forces affect the skin, providing the infant is well-nourished. All functions of the skin are intact; however, the functions are not well-developed, so the infant's skin needs to be protected.

During adolescence, the skin changes. As it matures, it is building resistance to environmental stresses, functioning at a better capacity as compared to infancy. As the skin changes for adulthood, there is a surge in sex hormones. The endogenous androgens cause the development of the sebaceous glands, hair follicular units, and apocrine glands. The sebaceous glands enlarge and accumulate lipids. With increased oil production, you may notice oilier skin and production of acne due to clogged pores. Vellus hairs (fine hairs) develop in certain areas that are influenced by the androgen hormone such as the upper lip, chin, sides of the face, chest, axillary areas, private areas, and legs. The apocrine gland enlarges and produces a particular scent or body odor. Again, as the years pass, the affected areas mature into adulthood, producing a stronger scent, coarse terminal hairs, and oil.

During the post-menopausal period, the sex hormones plummet in production. The skin becomes drier due to decreased oil production from the oil glands. Besides turning gray, hair production diminishes or stops altogether. Both the sweat glands and apocrine glands increase in activity. Women notice excessive sweating and a change in body odor. The skin becomes thin and not as firm due to lack of collagen production and loss of fat underneath the skin. There is the appearance of slack skin, which is due to a decrease in elastin production. Dryness with slack skin produces a sagging appearance of the eyelids, neck, jawline, cheeks, fine lines, and wrinkles. Jowls appear as well as permanent lines running from the tip of the nose to the corner of the mouth. There is a loss of cheeks. Wrinkles initially appearing only during smiles, frowning, or active muscle movement now become permanently present at rest. You also notice hollow and sunken lower eyelids. Age spots can form with benign growths, and the skin develops a darker pigment from being exposed to the sun for a number of years, not to mention the potential to develop pre-cancerous lesions or overt skin cancer. Women notice the development of bruising much easier. Unwanted hairs develop on the upper lip, chin, jawline, and there is diminished hair growth on the scalp.

Chapter 3

SKIN ENEMIES

There are several enemies of the skin with the sun being the greatest enemy of unprotected skin. The sun rays are comprised of ultraviolet A, B, and C. Ultraviolet C rays are the most dangerous; however, they are blocked by the earth's ozone layer. Ultraviolet A and B rays can both penetrate the earth's surface; however, ultraviolet B rays cause sunburn. Over time, with too much sun exposure, ultraviolet A and B rays can cause damage to the skin and sunburn. The sun causes the breakdown of collagen, increased pigment production, an increase in the appearance of wrinkles, and mottled coloration of the skin. It also causes an increase in the growth of benign lesions, both precancerous and cancerous. The sun also has benefits such as production of vitamin D that helps growing bones and teeth.

Another enemy is tobacco or cigarette smoking. Tobacco causes premature aging of the skin as seen with the formation of wrinkles. Tobacco contains thousands of substances that contribute to a number of problems for the skin. Nicotine causes narrowing of the blood vessels, carbon monoxide displacement of oxygen, leading to a decreased intake of oxygen and nutrients like vitamins A and C which causes increased dryness, uneven skin tone, sagging of the skin, and premature wrinkling. Decreased intake of vitamin C causes further damage to the collagen since decreased vitamin C leads to a decreased mechanism to protect and repair the skin damage. Toxins damage collagen and elastin, which typically keep the skin firm and supple. Tobacco also causes tooth loss, discoloration of teeth, and gum damage. Tobacco is the leading cause of oral cancers. Besides wrinkles on the face, tobacco also causes sagging skin on the face, arms, and breasts. Lines around the lips that are very hard to correct, age spots, and stains on the fingers and nails are common in tobacco users. Smokers experience an increase in skin conditions such as psoriasis and infections with the Human Papillomavirus. Wounds take longer to heal. Women notice an increase in stretch marks or a longer time for redness to fade along with increased fat around the organs.

One glass of red wine is healthy; however, more than that can cause increased inflammation in the skin. Inflammation damages the collagen, which leads to wrinkles and sagging skin. Also, alcohol is a mild diuretic. It causes dehydration, which causes dryness of the skin. Alcohol can also cause decreased absorption of vitamins and micronutrients leading to further changes of the skin, with the body losing important vitamins to help repair skin damage. You may also notice bloating and puffiness of the face. Also, hormonal disruption occurs due to the production of sugar from alcohol, which leads to a spike in insulin that suppresses the sex hormones. Suppression of sex hormones causes decrease in collagen formation, and thus, premature aging. Some skin conditions like rosacea are worse after alcohol intake. Clients notice increased broken blood vessels, redness, and sometimes acne production with increased alcohol intake. Other clients complained of breakouts with increased alcohol intake. Alcohol causes crystallized skin cells called glycation, leading to less plump, duller skin. Another skin conditions that can be affected by alcohol is eczema. Clients with eczema, after drinking too much alcohol, experience a disruption of the good bacteria in the gut, microbiomes, which leads to an alteration in the immune system that help control the outbreaks of their disease.

Eating a poor diet leads to missing nutrients for the skin. The loss of color or freshness and dryness with the inability to repair damaged cells all lead to premature aging. Lack of vitamins and micronutrients can cause the inability to repair damage to the skin, increasing premature aging.

Toxins released in the air cause free radical formation and therefore damage to the collagen. Again, damage to the collagen leads to an increase in premature aging of the skin.

Stress and lack of sleep often go hand-in-hand. Not enough sleep causes increased stress hormone release, which leads to inflammation causing collagen breakdown. Women notice swollen eyes, dark circles, or their faces appear dry. Stress destroys collagen. Together, they can both create a vicious cycle with lack of sleep leading to stress or stress leading to a lack of sleep.

Dry weather increases the appearance of wrinkles, whereas alcohol or medications along with insufficient water intake can all lead to a dry, dull complexion and obvious aging.

Overall, the skin does a good job of taking care of itself. Many skin problems occur from our lack of taking care of this large organ, but in some cases, we cause problems from doing too much to the skin. You start with one solution to a problem, then you develop another problem from the first solution. Another solution is needed for the second problem, and so forth. That's not to mention adding a procedure to the surmounting products that are applied to the skin. The ramifications of procedures done by a professional or your very own actions can produce permanent adverse outcomes to your skin.

Chapter 4

SKIN CHALLENGES

Have you noticed your face and arms? The majority of the time, the skin is two different shades. Certain areas are darker such as the area around the mouth as compared to the rest of your face or the front of your arms as compared to the back of your arms. The various shades of your skin tone could be due to increased exposure to sunlight in these areas. The increase in pigmentation could also be due to increased reactivity of the melanocytes. Regardless of the reason, it is programmed in your genes to have this varied shade of skin tone.

Discoloration can occur due to certain rashes. It is common for clients of ethnic skin to develop discoloration after a rash or eruption that occurs on the skin. Outbreaks of their disease increase such as eczema, atopic dermatitis, dermatitis, lichen planus, or any skin rash that disrupts the basal layer of the skin where the melanocytes are located. There is an increased risk for development of discoloration after the rash resolves, leaving a darker hue that requires lightening creams to diminish the discoloration.

Infections such as bacterial infections and some fungal infections such as ringworm are notorious for causing hyperpigmentation once the infection has resolved. With the landscape of a battlefield occurring between the infection and your body's arsenal, all the chemical warfare is released to eradicate the infection, leaving the destruction of war, scarring, discoloration, and hair loss if occurring in a hair-bearing area. The sooner the infection is identified and treated, the better the outcome with resolution of the organism and prevention or reversal of discoloration.

Mimickers of discoloration include vascular lesions or rashes that are vascular in nature that appear as discoloration. This is commonly seen in clients who present with rosacea, systemic lupus with the butterfly rash, or Erythema Ab Igne. Erythema Ab Igne is a condition when a heating device is applied closely to the skin for a duration of time and causes fishnet-like appearance of the dilated veins in the areas exposed to the heat source (either a heater or heating pad). In ethnic skin, the dilation of blood vessels appear hyperpigmented or violaceous color instead of red. In clients with darker skin tones, it is more difficult to distinguish redness from discoloration due to the increased melanocytic activity. Increased melanocytic activity causing increased pigmentation makes it harder for a physician to accurately diagnose the condition. Other factors and tools may be necessary to help diagnose a skin condition.

Injuries are common, ranging from nicks due to shaving, linear marks from scratching, or nodules from picking. Once the injury occurs, intentionally or by accident, the body sends inflammatory cells in the areas to start the healing process. The healing process includes inflammatory cells that release cytokines to kill any germs, increased blood flow, and increased collagen formation, among other factors of healing. Cytokines affect the melanocytes and cause an increase in pigmentation production along with loss of pigmentation in some areas due to scarring.

Other causes of discoloration include reactions to the sun along with certain chemicals on the skin causing a second-degree burn. This is commonly experienced by vacationers at sunny locations who perhaps spill a margarita on their sun-exposed skin and develop a second degree burn that later develops into discolored spots or linear markings resembling a spill. The name for this is Margarita Dermatitis. Furocoumarin is the chemical that reacts with the sun's rays causing the reaction, which leads to a second-degree burn and discoloration. This same reaction can occur with other furocoumarin containing fruits and vegetables such as carrots, celery, figs, wild dill, and citrus fruits like limes, lemons, grapefruits, or oranges.

Changes in the sex hormone level is the cause for the bilateral increased pigmentation commonly seen on the temple areas of the face, upper lip, or bilateral upper half of the face. Melasma is due to either increase or decrease in hormone levels such as pregnancy, alterations in birth control, hormone replacement, or hereditary causes.

Certain conditions cause decreased production of pigmentation, resulting in various shades of pigmentation or no production of pigment as seen in injuries, injections, and certain rashes. Reports of lighter areas can occur during or after the rash or infection resolves. As in the case of tinea versicolor, the infection can cause a decrease in melanocytic activity resulting in lighter spots. Once the infection is treated, the melanocytes resume production and the re-pigmentation occurs. Vitiligo is the result of the destruction of melanocytes. The outcome is patches or large areas of no pigment.

Heavy metals and medication can deposit in the epidermis or top layer of the skin, causing increased pigmentation. This can be seen not only in the skin but also in the oral mucosa. Oral medications that can cause increase pigmentation include NSAIDs like ibuprofen, phenytoin for seizures, antimalarial medications, amiodarone, antipsychotic drugs, cytotoxic drugs used for cancers, and oral antibiotics such as tetracycline or minocycline. Heavy metals including lead, mercury, silver, bismuth, arsenic, gold, excessive zinc, iron, and manganese can also cause increase pigmentation.

Chapter 5

SKIN HORMONES

Three sex hormones affect the skin: estrogen, progesterone, and testosterone. Other major hormones include cortisol and thyroid stimulating hormones. All of these hormones play a major role in the skin.

Estrogen is a major player for the skin. Estrogen increases collagen production, resulting in increased skin thickness and skin hydration. Estrogen helps with wound healing. It improves barrier function and causes increased redness in the skin. It increases skin hydration by boosting hyaluronic acid production, a naturally occurring carbohydrate present in the spaces between skin cells, where it provides moisture, plumpness, firmness, and suppleness to the skin.

A deficiency of estrogen, which occurs during menses, causes skin sensitivity. Low estrogen levels lead to an increase in sebum production by not having adequate amounts of estrogen to counteract the effects of testosterone on the skin. Therefore, testosterone causes an increase in oil production causing blockage resulting in acne. This same outcome of acne production can occur with the imbalance of progesterone with low estrogen. High progesterone and low estrogen cause behavioral changes leading to emotional eating and binge eating. The result is a spike in insulin levels and thus acne production. Besides outbreaks, decreased production of estrogen is associated with less collagen and elastin production. This decrease in estrogen production makes the skin thinner, and with less elastin produced, you will experience wrinkling and sagging of the skin.

There are several ways to correct the estrogen levels. Natural ways to increase estrogen levels include avoidance of high levels of stress, correct poor sleep cycles, and avoidance of irregular eating habits. Sickness can prevent the adrenal glands from producing more estrogen. Natural estrogen fluctuates in women in their mid to late 40s and eventually falls to very low levels thereafter. Correcting estrogen levels with synthetic estrogen such as ethinyl estradiol not only controls acne outbreaks by suppressing ovulation and androgen production, but it also maintains the skin's collagen, thickness, firmness, and ability to retain moisture.

Progesterone is the second most important sex hormone. Progesterone increases skin elasticity and circulation. A deficiency in progesterone causes wrinkles, sagging, and dull-looking skin. Treatment for decreased amounts of progesterone includes eating foods high in vitamin B6, which will increase progesterone levels while decreasing excessive levels of estrogen. Other treatments include eating foods high in zinc and maintaining your ideal body weight, since overweight individuals have an increase in estrogen. Exercising in moderation will increase progesterone levels, whereas excessive exercise can cause an increase in production and release in cortisone, which lowers the production of progesterone. Eating foods like soy and flaxseed, which cause increased estrogen levels can lead to an imbalance of progesterone and estrogen hormones. Progesterone levels decline with menopause as well as with stress. Therefore, stress management and sleeping well is crucial to maintaining healthy progesterone levels. Two percent natural progesterone creams (not FDA approved) can also help dry skin, wrinkling on the face, and brown spots on the hands and arms. Be careful with this product because it may cause irritation and PMS-like symptoms.

Lastly, testosterone causes increased oil production by increasing production of lipids in the sebaceous (oil) glands. This could be considered a good or bad situation for teenagers, women, or menopausal women. Too much oil production can lead to oily skin, clogged pores, and acne. We also see increased testosterone levels in women with polycystic ovarian syndrome. Testosterone at normal levels causes increased sebum production. Testosterone production tapers off in women around 40-50 years of age. Women experience no skin problems, whereas men experience dry skin. Replacement testosterone is used for other concerns such as decreased libido in women, but replacement therapy is not used or needed for the skin of women.

Cortisone, a steroid hormone, is the flight or fight hormone that increases during stress, helps defend the body, and causes increased radical formation in the skin. Cortisone levels rise with increased stress or lack of sleep. Prolonged elevated exogenous or endogenous cortisone levels can lead to acne-like eruptions, weight gain, destruction of collagen, sagging skin, and stretch marks. Getting proper sleep and controlling your stress levels can lead to the normalizing of cortisone levels. Decreasing or stopping exogenous cortisone can also normalize cortisone levels.

Excessive levels of thyroid hormone cause dull, dry skin, skin rashes, and brittle hair and nails. Low levels of thyroid hormone produce moist skin and thin hair. Replacement hormones such as levothyroxine normalize the underactive thyroid gland. Various treatments are used for an overactive thyroid gland such as radioactive iodine, surgery, and oral medications.

Chapter 6

SKIN PSYCHOLOGY

There are three types of psychodermatological disorders. The first is skin disorders that are affected by depression or other emotional states, for example acne or eczema. The second group are psychological problems that are caused by disfiguring skin disorders such as acne, alopecia, or hidradenitis suppurative. And last, there are psychiatric disorders that manifest themselves via the skin such as delusional parasitosis.

The reason skin problems can cause intense distress in individuals is because skin disorders are more obvious to onlookers as compared to hypertension or diabetes. Flare-ups of psoriasis, acne, and eczema are unpredictable, and people may have a psychological reaction that seems out of proportion to their actual skin conditions.

All of these conditions can leave a person feeling like they have no control of their skin disorders.

Severity of a dermatological disorder does not correlate with psychological impact. For example, nodulocystic acne upsets a person; however, it does not cause psychological distress, whereas another person with one acne bump attempts suicide.

People with skin disorders reported lowered self-esteem and self-confidence, anxiety, helplessness, and depression. Many of my clients with hidradenitis suppurativa reported that they avoid face-to-face contact when they have a skin disorder. They also noticed their tendencies to become secluded. They avoid gatherings and social functions with friends and family.

A vicious cycle of stress or depression and other psychological problems can make skin problems worse. Dermatologists may see that in clients with acne, rosacea, psoriasis, itching, eczema, pain, and hives. The good news is that treating psychological problems can also improve skin problems.

The goal of treatment is to restore the client's sense of control over their condition and their reactions to them. The number one way for that to occur is to see a professional to treat the skin problem. If a primary care provider has not been able to control the problem, seeing a dermatologist can save time by quickly diagnosing and treating the condition.

Give the skin condition time to resolve using a traditional dermatology regimen, hypnosis, or hypnotherapy. Hypnosis is a technique for putting a person in a state of high concentration on a single idea and a relaxed state of mind where the subject is more open to suggestions. People are awake or in a trance. Hypnosis can be used to change behaviors such as helping a person to stop smoking or lose weight through repetitive suggestions while in a trance. It can also be used to help people cope with anxiety, pain, and stress. Therapists put a person in a trance-like state with the use of mental imagery and soothing verbal repetition. Once in a trance-like state, clients' minds are open to positive messages.

Many of my clients are part of support groups, which are common on Facebook; however, support groups still meet in person. Support groups allow members to share their personal stories, so everyone can learn. There is a support group for many conditions such as alcoholism, hidradenitis suppurative, or the death of a loved one, to name a few. It helps to be in a group where everyone shares the same interests and many times the same experiences. You are able to share your feelings and get helpful information. Being part of a support group allows you to learn about yourself, help others, gain hope for your condition, and decrease anxiety. Support groups are free of charge.

Biofeedback is when a person is connected to electrodes on their skin and a monitoring box. The box monitors the subject's ability to control bodily involuntary actions. This is used to control stress and anxiety.

Meditation is another cognitive treatment modality used to control your reaction. You focus on breathing techniques in a relaxed state. Meditation centers a person, allowing them to regroup. You may notice an increased ability to control your emotions and your response to stressful situations. Meditation also increases endorphins that improve sleep, thus aiding in the control of stress.

Guided imagery allows you to visualize yourself being or appearing the way you desire. Practicing visual imagery keeps the goal in your conscious thought process and thus, one can make positive changes by staying focused.

Progressive muscle relaxation helps with stress and controls your emotional responses to adverse situations. While relaxing, you focus concentration on contracting each muscle group in a systematic way. Total concentration reminds you to practice self-control, reminding the individual that they have control over any situation. Progressive muscle relaxation causes increased release of endorphins, the feel-good hormone.

Cognitive-behavior therapy helps the person manage stress. By recognizing the behavior, you can learn tools to better control the response. Cognitive-behavior therapy is led by a therapist who gives feedback.

If the techniques above do not help to alleviate stress, then seeing a psychologist will be beneficial. Since there are times when skin problems are an outward manifestation of an underlying mental disorder, a psychologist will be able to diagnose the condition. For example, attention-deficit disorder or obsessive-compulsive disorder may be diagnosed if the client picks their skin.

Chapter 7

SKIN CARE

Keeping everyday skin care simple is the take home message. Many problems women have with their skin is from doing too much. Only use what you need to achieve beautiful skin. What may work for your friend may not work for you. When purchasing a new product, try a low concentration first to make sure you can tolerate the ingredients before going to a stronger concentration. Always use the product for at least three days before adding a new product to your skincare regimen. If you develop a skin rash or irritation from a product, you will be able to identify which product is the causative agent. Use the product for the recommended amount of time before stopping because you did not see results based on your timeline. I instruct my clients on the amount of time it takes to see results for each product they purchase, so they will not stop using the product because they did not see results in two days when it will take approximately two weeks to see results.

The goal of products applied to the skin is to alleviate the concerns. Common diagnoses I've seen over the years for products applied to the skin are irritant dermatitis or contact dermatitis. Both present as a rash in the areas of product application. Irritant dermatitis can be seen immediately from the first day of application or up to three to five days after use. Clients have complained of burning of the skin, sensitivity, and sometimes itching and peeling. The skin can appear raw and red with a glistening surface. There may be weeping of the skin with crusting formation for acute cases. Besides using a product that causes irritation to your skin, aggressive exfoliation, either mechanical or chemical, can remove the protective layer of the skin, or the weeping and repetitive drying cycle can cause loss of the lipids in the skin. If weeping is present, it is due to the body's natural way of rinsing off the causative agent that is irritating the skin.

Treatment includes discontinuing the offending agent. Even if the area was an acne-prone location, the most important thing is to clear the new rash fast and restore the protective barrier. Once that has been achieved, you can return to clearing your skin of the initial skin problem. If you can use a lower concentration of the same product, you can try it but only after the skin has returned to baseline. After stopping the product, rinse the area with warm water and apply a mild ointment-based steroid since it will not contain preservatives that are alcohol-based in nature. Apply the ointment twice a day for about one to two weeks. Thereafter, use a moisturizer that contains ceramides to restore the lipid layer. Once the skin has cleared, a new product can be tried.

Allergic contact dermatitis is when the skin is allergic to the offending product, meaning the skin was exposed to the product in the past and developed a mild reaction, but on reuse of the same product, the patient is experiencing a significant rash that presents as blister formation or dry, itchy, red eruptions in the area of application. Again, stop using the offending agent. Lance the blister with a sterile needle, clean the skin to remove the offending product, and apply a mid-strength steroid that is either a cream, lotion, foam, or gel. The skin is usually intact except for the lanced blister; therefore, steroids containing, alcohol-based preservatives like creams, lotions, foams, or gels are safe to use and will penetrate the areas faster than ointments. The more wet the areas are, the more drying the steroid should be. If several blisters are present, gels containing steroids will clear the skin faster, whereas if they are just red, itchy eruptions, a cream or lotion will work well. After the resolution of the rash, make a note to self and any other physician that you are allergic to that particular product, so it will not be prescribed again.

Wash the face with a clean cloth daily and rub in a circular motion on the central face but on the lower neck and lower cheeks, rub upwards against gravity. Either bar soap or liquid cleansers are good to use. A basic, gentle cleanser without harsh chemicals works well for most. If your skin is very dry, a moisturizing cleanser is best. For oily skin or skin with comedonal acne, a cleanser containing salicylic or glycolic acid works best to control oil production. Glycolic acid is a more elegant and expensive ingredient than salicylic acid; therefore, it is common to find glycolic acid ingredients in anti-aging products sold in doctor offices or spas, whereas salicylic acid ingredients are found in acne products sold in retail stores, doctor offices, and spas. Exfoliators are sold in various concentrations. When used with other drying products, purchase a low strength exfoliating cleanser before increasing the strength to make sure it does not cause dryness or irritation. Cleansers containing benzoyl peroxide are used to help control acne outbreaks. Benzoyl peroxide has antimicrobial properties to help clear acne. It is sold in different strengths from 2 percent to 10 percent. Since it can irritate and dry the skin, I recommend starting with a low concentration and gradually increasing the strength on the next purchase. Benzoyl peroxide also has bleaching properties. It is common to notice bleaching of your colored towels, pillowcases, or collars on your tops if you use benzoyl peroxide cleansers daily. Black soap is a mild product to cleanse the skin. You can cleanse the face daily or up to three times a day depending on your activity level. Once to twice a day is standard to cleanse the face. Women who wear cosmetics are advised to remove the make-up and wash the face again. Athletes may need to wash their faces two to three times a day to keep the face clean after training or games.

A cleanser should be gentle on the skin. Adverse effects from cleansers may not occur until after a few days of use. Use the new product for a few days before adding new skin care products to your skin regimen making sure you do not have any adverse reactions such as irritation or an allergic reaction.

Toners are used to restore the skin's pH. After washing, apply the toner during the morning. There are three grades of toners, with rosewater being the mildest and witch hazel being more astringent. It is very important to make sure the toner is not strong since by definition, an astringent dries the cells of fluid. If you are using a retinoid at night and notice irritation or dry skin during the day, do not use a toner.

Moisturizers can range in various textures. The goal is to find a moisturizer that satisfies the feel you desire, while moisturizing your skin and not clogging your pores. Moisturizers can contain sunscreens or exfoliators. Again, choose the product that feels good to your skin. Sunscreens that are in moisturizers do not last all day. Usually the ingredients are not water-proof or sweat resistant, thus they last less than one hour. Reapplication is necessary to prevent sun burn. If you develop acne, choose moisturizers that are non-comedogenic, which means it does not clog your pores. Exfoliators are products that peel the top layer of skin microscopy to release any contents of whiteheads and/or blackheads. Exfoliators include salicylic acid or glycolic acid in various strengths. Again, start mild and increase in strength on the next purchase.

I put hyaluronic acid after moisturizers because I have my clients use it as a hydrator with a moisturizer or alone as a hydrator. Hyaluronic acid is a product that our bodies make naturally. It gives our skin the youthful appearance by keeping the skin plump-looking, thicker, and supple. As we age, our bodies gradually decrease the production of hyaluronic acid. During aging, you will notice increased wrinkle formation and shallowness of the skin. After application of hyaluronic acid, you notice immediate diminishing of fine wrinkles and increasing plumpness of the skin. The effects last a day; therefore, reapplication is a must. For my clients who have an oily complexion and desire a moisturizer, I use hyaluronic acid to dilute the oil and provide hydration.

Exfoliators are used to keep the skin youthful. Prescription exfoliators include prescription grade retinoids containing products, whereas over-the-counter exfoliators include salicylic acid, alpha hydroxy acid, glycolic acid, lactic acids, and non-retinol, non-prescription grade retinoids. They peel the skin in a microscopic fashion. You should not have major peeling when using these products. It does not indicate the product is too strong, but the majority of women do not want their faces peeling while in public. Initially, peeling can occur for the first two weeks, but thereafter if it has not subsided, I recommend decreasing the strength. Many exfoliators have several strengths. Just know the strength that works for you may not work for someone else. After washing and patting your face dry, apply a pea-sized amount on your finger. Dab the pea-sized amount all over your face, avoiding the eyelids, sides of the eyes, nose, and lips. Rub the exfoliator into the skin. Prescription grade exfoliators are usually applied at night, whereas non-prescription grade exfoliators can be applied during the day and at night. Prescription grade exfoliators and retinoids not only cause peeling of the skin, but formation of hyaluronic acid, diminishes fine lines and wrinkles, evens out skin tone, smooths the texture of the skin, tightens the pores, and by removing dead skin, causes a subtle glow. While using an exfoliator, peeling can be controlled by decreasing the concentration of the exfoliator, or you can use the same strength and add a moisturizer to the skin after the application of the exfoliator. Be careful not to use an exfoliator that causes severe irritation to the skin.

Sunscreen is the protection that is needed from the sun. It prevents the skin from aging prematurely. It can be a sunblock or sunscreen. Sunblock is a physical block that prevents the sun rays from interacting with the skin. The sunblock does not react with the skin, whereas sunscreens are chemicals that interact with the skin to provide protection from ultraviolet A and ultraviolet B rays. Physical blocks include titanium dioxide or zinc oxide, whereas sunscreens are various chemicals. Ultraviolet B rays are associated with sunburns, and both ultraviolet A and ultraviolet B rays are associated with the development of skin cancers. Sun Protection Factor (SPF) rates the blockage of ultraviolet B rays from the sun. To block sunrays, purchase a broad-spectrum sunscreen that covers both UVA and UVB rays.

Recommendations include purchasing sunscreen SPF30, which blocks about 97 percent of UVB after ten minutes exposure to the sun. Darker skin types can use sunscreen of SPF15 since they produce more melanin, which also acts as a protector against the sun. Sunscreen SPF15 blocks 93 percent of sun rays, SPF 30 blocks about 97 percent, and sunscreen SPF50 blocks about 98 percent. No sunscreen blocks 100 percent of sun rays; however, if a person has a history of skin cancers, I recommend sunscreen with at least an SPF50. There is only a 5 percent difference between sunscreens with SPF15 versus SPF50. However, for a person with a history of skin cancers is important. Sunscreens are sold in many formulations: sprays, gels, creams, lotions, and foams. Sunscreens are usually applied last in association with your skin regimen. However, they are applied underneath make-up. Some make-up has sunscreens in the product; however, it does not provide protection all day. Sunscreen should be reapplied every two to three hours as long as you are in the sun. If swimming, it should be reapplied once out of the pool. Purchase water resistant or waterproof products because these types of sunscreens last longer than the typical sunscreen. There are clothes that are available for purchase that are sun protective.

It has been proven that getting proper rest helps every organ of the body. Proper sleep allows the body, including the skin, time to repair itself. Sleeping at least seven hours causes you to be sensitive to the stress hormone, so the body will decrease production, thus decreasing inflammation of the skin. Blood flow increases in the skin to help rebuild itself and provide nutrients and oxygen.

Hydrating the skin is essential. Drinking plenty of water is elementary for the well-being of the body including the skin. Drinking water helps in circulation, digestion, excretion, and secretion, all of which contribute to the wellness and proper functioning of the body as well as the skin. Drinking at least eight cups a day for an average weight person is adequate. Water keeps the skin supple and radiant.

Chapter 8

SKIN HEALTH

EXERCISE

Exercise has profound positive effects on the skin. It keeps the skin healthy and vibrant. It increases blood flow, which increases the supply of oxygen to the skin that nourishes the skin cells by carrying nutrients to repair the damage from the sun and environment. Collagen production is increased by the increased activity of fibroblasts, which are cells that make collagen. It cleanses the skin by removing cellular debris out of the system. It decreases stress by decreasing the stress hormone, cortisone, and by releasing endorphins and regulating sex hormones, which aid in a better quality of sleep. During continuous stressful events, cortisone levels are elevated and saturate the cortisone cellular receptors. The high levels blunt the fluctuations in cortisol levels, and more cortisone will need to be released to gain the desired effects. The elevated cortisol levels diminish the sensitivity of the adrenal gland. Thus the adrenal gland needs a more stressful situation to release an elevated amount of hormone to produce the same effect. This leaves you mentally wound up at night with the inability to sleep. However, when you exercise in moderation, not only does it alleviate stress, but it sends a signal to the adrenal glands to normalize cortisol production. Getting enough exercise improves sleep. Exercise decreases the body's blood sugar more effectively and decreases insulin levels thereby diminishing outbreaks on the skin. It decreases inflammation of the entire body leading to decreased free radical damage. Self-confidence and self-worth improve with physical changes and overall health. Self-worth increases before skin problems improve. Exercise decreases stress and anxiety. Exercise helps with fighting infections by increasing immunity and detoxification. The muscle contractions help the lymphatic system. Visceral fat around the organs causes low grade inflammation. It is linked to diabetes, heart disease, and breast cancer. Visceral fat can cause an increase in estrogen hormones that leads to an imbalance of sex hormones. Exercising regularly causes the body to increase in organelles to burn the fat more efficiently. Endorphins, testosterone, and human growth hormones all improve the appearance of hair, skin, and muscle tone. Cardiovascular exercise is recommended five days a week for thirty minutes, and strength training to increase tone and burn fat faster is recommended three days a week.

NUTRITION

Foods, vitamins, and supplements are needed to help the skin look its best. Fatty fish elevated in omega 3 fatty acids helps the skin by increasing the thickness, suppleness, and moisturization. Deficiency causes dry skin. Omega 3, found in salmon, also reduces inflammation, helping reduce redness and acne. This is also a good source of vitamin E, which is an antioxidant. Fatty fish contains zinc, which fights inflammation and keeps the skin tight.

Avocados are another food that is good for the skin. Avocados contain high doses of vitamin E and vitamin C. Vitamin E is an antioxidant that becomes more effective when combined with vitamin C. Vitamin C creates collagen, which keeps the skin strong. When vitamin C levels are decreased, you notice roughness, dryness, and scaly skin with the tendency to bruise easily. Vitamin C protects the skin from oxidative damage.

Brussels sprouts contain large amounts of vitamin C. Vitamin C is also found in red peppers, blueberries, and citrus fruits. Vitamin C makes collagen act as an antioxidant.

Walnuts are another beneficial food. It contains Omega 3 and Omega 6 along with a significant amount of selenium. Selenium neutralizes free radical production that damages the skin.

Sweet potatoes have significant levels of beta carotene, which is classified as a carotenoid and acts as a natural sun blocker and anti-inflammatory food. It protects your skin cells from sun exposure, prevents sunburn, cell death, and dry, wrinkled skin. Appropriate amounts will give the skin a warm, orange color, causing an overall healthier appearance to the skin. Large quantities of carotenoid will cause a yellowish orange discoloration of the skin.

Broccoli is another notable vegetable that is good for the skin. It contains sulforaphane. Sulforaphane is a compound that has anti-cancer properties. It protects the skin against sun damage by neutralizing free radicals and switching on the other protective systems. By providing protection, it decreases the number of skin cells killed by ultraviolet light.

Soy is an isoflavone. An isoflavone is known to mimic or block estrogen in our bodies. Eating soy daily will cause a decrease in fine wrinkles and improve skin elasticity. It improves skin dryness and increases collagen formation. It also helps protect the skin from ultraviolet damage.

Dark chocolate should contain at least 70 percent cocoa to be considered beneficial. Cocoa is good for the skin both orally and topically. It fights free radical formation and softens and detoxifies the skin. Internally, it increases blood flow and makes new cells.

Green tea, containing catechins, provides antioxidant properties to protect the skin from sun damage. Green tea decreases redness, improves moisture of the skin, diminishes roughness, and promotes thickness and elasticity of the skin. Not to mention, it creates mental alertness.

Resveratrol is found in red wine. The product is found in the skin of red grapes. Anthocyanins, which gives the grapes their skin color, is an antioxidant such as resveratrol. Both slow down the aging process and repair the damage that free radicals create.

VITAMINS

Vitamins are important to the functioning of the skin. Vitamin A, a retinoid, causes exfoliation of the skin if applied topically and is used to reverse aging. It functions as an antioxidant when taken orally; however, when used topically, it is an exfoliator. Vitamin C, a water-soluble vitamin, helps produce collagen. Vitamin C, when applied topically, is used to even out the skin tone. It is an excellent alternative to hydroquinone that is used to bleach the skin. Vitamin D is the "sunshine" vitamin. It fights infections. Vitamin D also provides energy: however, if you keep your skin covered, you may need replacement vitamin D. Vitamin E has antioxidant properties. Vitamin E helps diminish fine lines and wrinkles. Vitamin K helps with wound healing and diminishes bruising, dark circles around the eyes, spider veins, stretch marks, and scars. Vitamin B3, or niacin or niacinamide, not only decreases the appearance of aging skin but also brightens the skin. Vitamin B5, or pantothenic acid or panthenol, prevents water loss. It is found in many topical products for the skin and in products for the hair.

Other trace minerals that are good for the skin includes selenium that neutralizes free radical production and skin aging. Choline helps with the integrity of the skin cell membrane. Folic acid helps with inflammation and increases collagen production to diminish aging skin. CoQ10 is a phytonutrient that cleanses the skin of free radical production and reduces the formation of sagging and wrinkled skin. Hyaluronic acid exhibits moisture retaining properties when taken internally. When topically applied, it is readily absorbed resulting in plump, hydrated skin with diminished wrinkles.

Chapter 9

SKIN PRODUCTS

There are many products to choose from when it comes to skin products. The majority has the same ingredients with different bases. Others have combined ingredients. When choosing all-natural ingredients, more time is needed before you may see an outcome as compared to products that have natural and man-made ingredients. Regardless, all the products serve to clear the skin. It is a matter of personal preference and how well it works. The three major categories of skin care products are: anti-aging, anti-acne, and discoloration. Skin care products mentioned in the everyday skin care chapter should be included in your daily regimen for all skin types.

Anti-aging skin care products include hyaluronic acid, COQ10, retinoids, exfoliators, sunscreens, vitamins D, E and K, collagen, and peptides. Anti-aging products repair the damage caused by ultraviolet rays and pollution either by evening out the skin tone, preventing wrinkles, diminishing wrinkles, and/or tightening pores. Since hyaluronic acid naturally diminishes as we age, applying this product daily temporarily helps to diminish the visible signs of aging.

Hyaluronic acid, as stated in Chapter 4, can be used in place of a moisturizer or along with a moisturizer. Since the production diminishes as we age, replacement as a topical agent is temporary with no long-term effects. Tretinoin increases the production of hyaluronic acid. Even though the effects of hyaluronic acid are temporary with daily application, you can use hyaluronic acid until tretinoin increases the production of hyaluronic acid. The anti-aging changes that occur with tretinoin are present for a prolonged period of time.

Coenzyme Q10, CoQ10, is an antioxidant that can be taken orally or applied to the skin. As an antioxidant, it removes the free radicals that were formed in the skin from pollutants or sun exposure. COQ10 is found throughout the body in the heart, kidneys, pancreas, and liver. Low levels of COQ10 causes problems. In the heart, low levels of COQ10 has been linked to congestive heart failure and cardiovascular disease. Low levels of COQ10 has been linked to fibromyalgia, polycystic ovary disease, and the formation of wrinkles in the skin. When taking COQ10 supplements, you will experience repair and disappearance of fine lines and wrinkles in six months.

Retinoids stimulate the production of collagen, hyaluronic acid, and elastin, which reduces visible wrinkles and large pores, controls acne, and fades hyperpigmentation. It takes time to see all the changes. Retinoids are applied at night before bed. A moisturizer can be applied over the retinoid if the area is dry.

Exfoliators, as mentioned previously in Chapter 4, promote facial rejuvenation by removing dead cells. You can exfoliate mechanically (same as physically) or chemically. Mechanical (physical) exfoliators include sponges that have an abrasive side yet are gentle to use on the skin and natural products such as sugar scrubs or pumice stones. Chemical exfoliators include retinoids, non-retinoid exfoliators, and chemical peels. For mechanical exfoliators, apply the product to clean, wet skin and rub constantly, then rinse off after one to two minutes. This can be repeated two to three times a week.

Sunscreens are considered a basic product that should be used daily, also mentioned in Chapter 4. The problem is not that sunscreens are not used, but they're not used regularly with application every two to three hours. Blocking UVA and UVB rays prevents further sun damage.

Vitamins A, D, E, K, C, B3, and B5 are mixed with other anti-aging creams to provide a natural approach to skin care. All have an antioxidant effect to repair the skin from free radical attacks, help with discoloration, skin healing, and water retention.

Collagen ingestion can increase collagen production and improve elasticity. Collagen supplements and drinks can also improve skin hydration. Collagen is a large molecule; therefore, the hydrolyzed collagen or collagen peptides is a low weight molecule. Peptides are new in the anti-aging arena; they provide amino acids for your body to produce collagen. Collagen not only helps your skin but also helps your joints. It increases bone density and muscle mass. Collagen supplements decrease joint pain by increasing muscle and tendon mass, thus helping stabilize the joints. Collagen supplements help with weight loss by increasing muscle mass with added exercise, so your body burns more fat. It helps your hair by allowing your hair to absorb more dye or provides structural protection if using chemicals on the hairs. The powder form of collagen is used to make smoothies or shakes. Collagen supplements are manufactured from shellfish, shark cartilage, beef, pigs, or eggs. If you are allergic to any of these products, I do not recommend collagen, especially if you are not able to identify the source of the collagen supplements you purchase. Other ways to obtain collagen internally besides collagen supplements is through your diet. Foods that create the environment to help make collagen include soy bioflavonoids; beans make hyaluronic acid; dark leafy vegetables and prunes, the number one fruit high in antioxidant capabilities; blueberries; and red vegetables that are high in antioxidants; vitamin C, which is needed to make collagen found in citric fruits; and omega-3 fatty acid. Berries, cashews, and garlic, which increase sulfur content are products that can be used to increase collagen. When topically applied, collagen can be irritating for some people; it's not common but can occur. Any person taking calcium supplements along with collagen, especially if the collagen supplements are from marine life, can cause elevated calcium in the body. Elevated calcium can cause nausea, vomiting, constipation, joint pain, and cardiac arrhythmias. I recommend getting calcium levels checked if taking calcium supplements and hydrolyzed collagen supplements. Topically applied, collagen can cause dermatitis or irritation to the skin.

Products used to diminish blemishes and restore even skin are hydroquinone, kojic acid, tranexamic acid, glutathione, and vitamin C. All the products affect the melanocytes in the top layer of the skin and melasma in the dermal aspect of the skin.

Hydroquinone has been used for years to treat hyperpigmentation and melasma. It is the golden standard for comparison. It varies in concentration from 2 percent up to 12 percent with common concentrations of 2-3 percent as an over-the-counter product, 4 percent prescription filled at a retail pharmacy, and prescriptions of higher concentration are filled at apothecary pharmacies. It works by inhibiting the production of melanin (pigment). At high concentrations, it can cause irritation. Hydroquinone is applied twice a day unless it is mixed with a retinoid. If hydroquinone is mixed with a retinoid, it is only applied at night. Give it three months before determining whether it's working. A condition in which your skin turns a blue-black color called exogenous ochronosis appearing after prolonged use of hydroquinone at high concentrations can occur.

Kojic acid is made by fungi and is a byproduct of the fermentation of malting rice. Kojic acid is an over-the-counter product that inhibits the formation of melanin. Its concentration is in the range 1 to 4 percent. To avoid irritation, the recommendation is to stay at 2 percent or less. Kojic acid is applied twice a day except when mixed with an exfoliator such as glycolic acid. A compound of kojic acid and glycolic acid is applied at night. Kojic acid can be applied as a powder, serum, cream, or soap. Kojic acid in a higher concentration is mixed with glutathione as a soap to help lighten the unwanted dark areas.

Tranexamic acid can be taken orally, 325 mg tablets twice a day for eight to twelve weeks, applied as a 2 percent cream, or injected through microinjections in the skin. In all cases, tranexamic acid has performed well with outcomes just as good as hydroquinone mixed with dexamethasone, a steroid cream to stop inflammation and the burning sensation of hydroquinone. Tranexamic acid is a medication that is used to stop bleeding in women with prolonged bleeding problems. One side effect when taken orally is hypomenorrhea. Tranexamic acid cleared the discoloration due to increased pigmentation and melasma as well as freckles after three months and prevented the reoccurrence of pigmentation and freckles. Tranexamic acid is also used to treat rosacea. There are no studies that have reported absorption of microinjection of tranexamic acid into the skin. This medication is contraindicated in patients with a history of cardiovascular disease and clotting problems such as deep venous thrombosis (DVT) or pulmonary embolism (PE).

Glutathione is produced by the liver. It is found in fruits, vegetables, and meats. It is an antioxidant that boosts the immune system. It is used to lighten the skin by causing the melanin to lighten in color. It is administered through intravenous injections to produce the desired effects. Glutathione cream 2 percent can be used two times a day for ten weeks. Oral glutathione 500 mg taken twice a day for four weeks or intravenous injections of 1200 mg given twice weekly for eight weeks can be used with good success in lightening the skin.

Vitamin C brightens the dark spots. Vitamin C inhibits melanin production. It evens the skin tone after six months of applying twice a day. Using a retinoid at night with vitamin C shortens the duration time.

Chapter 10

SKIN PROCEDURES

Many procedures are available to help with clearing the skin, evening the skin tone, or just diminishing the signs of aging. Many require an experienced professional while others require machinery used by an experienced professional.

Facials consist of cleansing the face, dilating the pores with a steamer, massaging the face, and applying the necessary products to achieve the goal of customizing the facial to either provide extractions, deep pore cleansing, or basic facial. Extraction is the technique of removing comedones by using a noninvasive tool to release the contents of oil in the clogged pores. A deep pore cleansing facial includes using an enzyme to soften the contents deep in the skin pores. A deep pore cleansing facial helps remove the infected red papules on the face due to acne. After cleaning the dilated pores, the skin is cooled to allow the skin to return to baseline but with faster clearing of the inflammatory acne eruption and prevention of scarring. Over time, one will notice supple, clear skin and diminished blemishes. Pores are tight, skin looks rejuvenated, and the client feels good about themselves. I recommend monthly facials with customization of the facial depending on the month. If one month you present with eruptions on the face, I recommend a deep pore cleansing facial. If the next month there are comedones on the face, I recommend facials with extractions. If no eruptions are present, I recommend a basic facial to keep the pores tight. Facials can also be combined with chemical peels to help clear any discoloration.

Chemical peels involve different strengths of acids that cause aggressive exfoliation of the skin by dissolving the cement between the cells. Alpha hydroxy acid peels include glycolic acid, lactic acid, whereas beta hydroxy acid peels include salicylic acid. After washing the face, the acid is applied to the desired area and neutralized with water. The peel is left on the skin anywhere from three to five minutes. Stop rinsing the treated area with water once the stinging resolves. The treated areas may turn mildly pink or red depending on the person and the strength of the peel. Peeling can occur anywhere from one to three days after. I recommend using a bland moisturizer at night to counteract the excessive peeling. This type of peel is good for increased pigmentation, acne, or facial rejuvenation. Glycolic acid peels are performed every two weeks for resolution of discoloration and monthly for facial rejuvenation.

Trichloroacetic Acid (TCA) causes a deeper peel. It is tolerated in lighter skinned individuals. Once applied, it causes a frosting of the top layer of skin. It is rinsed off after three to five minutes. Water neutralizes the areas with resultant disappearance of the white coloration of the epidermis and minimization of redness. Trichloroacetic acid not only treats acne but also provides facial rejuvenation, improves melasma, fine lines, and wrinkles, sun damage, and precancerous growths. TCA peels can be performed monthly. Adverse effects of chemical peels include irritation or burning of the skin. Irritation or burning of the skin can occur if one does not stop their exfoliating products prior to a chemical peel, the chemical peel is left on the area too long, or the chemical peel is not neutralized. If irritation or chemical burn occurs, treatment includes rinsing the area(s), application of a mild steroid cream or ointment until the sensitivity has resolved, and correction of the discoloration if any occurs.

Microdermabrasion is gentle like a mild grade chemical peel. It uses salt crystals that can be cut for a coarser feel when treating the skin. It shoots salt crystals on the treated area and sucks it back into a waste container, leaving the skin smoother. Treatments are performed monthly. It causes remodeling of the skin after four to six treatments. Once completed, the skin may appear slightly swollen; however, there is no color change. Microdermabrasion can be used to treat acne and acne scarring, discoloration, mild scarring, and facial rejuvenation. Like any other exfoliator, microdermabrasion can cause irritation or abrasion if performed on skin that had other exfoliators applied and not discontinued in ample time or if the technique was performed in one area too long. Treatment consists of using a mild moisturizer or ointment-based product to protect the skin until the skin repairs itself.

Dermaplaning involves holding a blade perpendicular to the skin and scraping across the skin causing exfoliation. This technique helps remove fine vellus hairs; however, it is not recommended for active inflammatory acne eruptions. It should be performed monthly. Like any other exfoliation procedure, avoid irritating products or alcohol containing products after dermaplaning.

Microneedling or rollers cause microscopic injury to the skin with small needles. A roller uses the smallest set of needles evenly spaced, causing minimal injury as compared to microneedling. Rollers can be performed at home. Microneedling involves an experienced professional such as an esthetician who holds a hand-held motorized device to deliver pinpoint deeper placed injury on the desired locations. An anesthetic is applied before the process begins. The treated area causes formation of new skin, resulting in tighter and firmer skin and smaller pore size. It minimizes acne scarring and helps clear discoloration. It can be used with topical tranexamic acid to help alleviate unwanted areas of hyperpigmentation. After the microneedling is performed, tranexamic acid is applied over the skin.

To increase the effects of facial rejuvenation, platelet rich plasma (PRP) is applied to the exposed skin. Another name for this is a vampire facial. After microneedling, blood is drawn from the client's arm and centrifuged to separate the plasma and platelets from the red blood cells. The serum is applied to the microneedled skin. If microneedling is not performed, PRP can be injected directed into the skin. The growth factor in the serum penetrates the skin and improves the healing process, resulting in a better outcome as compared to just microneedling.

Botulinum toxin type A injections, a popular non-surgical cosmetic procedure, is used to soften if not totally block the formation of wrinkles on the face and neck. Botulinum toxin type A is a purified toxin made from a bacterium, *Clostridium botulinum*, which is used to block muscle movement. Botulinum toxin is used to reduce fine lines and wrinkles by paralyzing the underlying muscles. Not only is Botulinum toxin type A used to diminish wrinkles, but it is also used to treat hyperhidrosis, excessive sweating, migraines, muscle disorders, and some bladder and bowel disorders. Botulinum toxin type A can be injected in the forehead, glabella area, lateral sides of the eyes (crow's feet), upper lip, sides of the nose, chin, lower aspect of the jawline, and neck. A certain number of units is injected in the desired areas to paralyze the muscle thus blocking muscle movement and the formation of wrinkles. Botulinum toxin type A injections has a two-fold outcome. The initial outcome is the blockage of wrinkle formation which occurs within one day to two weeks after injection. The second outcome is the disappearance of wrinkles that are present at rest when there is no facial movement. The second outcome is achieved after Botulinum toxin type A injections have been consistently injected for approximately eighteen months in the same location. Botox is normally injected every two to four months depending on how fast the body breaks down the toxin. After cleaning the area, the desired location is injected with the appropriate amount of toxin. It is recommended to not lie down for up to four hours after treatment. Options of botulinum toxin type A include Botox®, Dysport®, Xeomin®, and Jeuveau.

Dermal fillers are injectable products that fill the diminished volume of soft tissue under the skin. Dermal fillers improve the appearance of aging, wrinkling, and sagging areas by filling in creases and lines, plumping up the lips and cheeks, and enhancing facial contours. Synthetic or natural dermal fillers are available as options. There are several products used to achieve a particular outcome. Depending on the location, the physician will make recommendations. The number of injections and the depth of insertion depend on the particular dermal filler chosen. There is minimal pain involved, with some of the fillers having anesthetic mixed into the product. There are three major groups of fillers used: 1. Hyaluronic acid containing filler; 2. calcium hydroxyapatite gel microspheres, which are made up of phosphate and calcium, which stimulates collagen production, and 3. poly-L-lactic acid, a synthetic dermal filler that also stimulates collagen production. Both hyaluronic acid and calcium hydroxyapatite gel microspheres dermal fillers are made naturally in our bodies. Hyaluronic acid containing dermal fillers vary in thickness by crosslinking the hyaluronic acid molecule, thus the duration of the effects once injected into the skin, can last anywhere from three months to twelve months. Hyaluronic acid containing fillers are injected in the lips, underneath the eyes, nasolabial fold (line from side of nose to corners of mouth), and cheeks. Calcium hydroxyapatite gel microspheres are thicker, and the effects last between twelve months to eighteen months. Calcium hydroxyapatite gel microspheres last longer because it stimulates collagen production. This product can be injected in the nasolabial fold, cheeks, scars, and dorsal hands. Poly-L-lactic acid, a synthetic filler offers longer lasting results, up to two years. Results are not present immediately like hyaluronic acid or calcium hydroxyapatite gel containing dermal fillers. It may take weeks before the results of the product are visible. However, since it is synthetic, it is recommended that you have an allergy test prior to treatment to make sure it will not cause a reaction. Poly-L-lactic acid is injected in the nasolabial fold areas or cheeks. Regardless of which product is used, once the area to be treated is cleaned and the dermal filler is injected, you will be able to resume normal activities immediately. You may need to postpone more strenuous activities for a day or two. Problems that can occur with fillers include not using enough to achieve the desired results, placement of the filler in the wrong location of the skin, or putting too thick of a filler in an area where lower molecular weight filler should be injected such as injecting a calcium hydroxyapatite gel filler in the lips. Another rare adverse effect is experiencing an allergic reaction to the filler.

Lasers are other procedures that can help the acne-prone or aging face. Intense Pulsed Light therapy gets rid of brown age spots and helps with clearing melasma. For dark-skinned individuals, the setting to treat melasma is very low to avoid burning the skin. Improvement is seen after one treatment. For age spots, treatments are performed monthly for four treatments, whereas for melasma, treatment is performed as needed.

Laser hair removal is safe in women of color with the use of the ND:YAG laser, which stands for yttrium aluminum garnet, a crystal that transmits light. All skin tones can be treated with this laser without concern of scarring. The areas can be treated every six to eight weeks. After six treatments, you will notice finer, lighter, or diminished hair growth. The laser is colorblind; therefore, only naturally colored hairs can be treated.

Non-ablative lasers are lasers that do not disrupt the integrity of the skin. The lasers cause the highest grade of facial rejuvenation as compared to other procedures that do not cause bleeding. Treatments are performed based on the protocol of the laser. This group of lasers are safe for all skin tones. The results are appreciated as late as six months after the last treatment. This helps with baseline redness, acne, scarring, dilated pores, and texture. Adverse effects can occur with the laser if products such as vitamin C containing products or retinoids are not stopped prior to having the procedure performed, makeup or other products are not removed from your skin prior to treatment, or the setting of the laser is too high.

Vascular lasers are used to alter vascular lesions such as broken blood vessels on the face and legs and red lesions scattered on the body. Lighter skin ethnic women would benefit from this treatment, whereas if darker skinned women have this procedure performed, they may experience a loss of pigment for up to one year.

Ablative lasers take off the top layer of skin (CO_2 laser) or cause significant disruption of skin integrity resulting in bleeding and injury. This procedure is not indicated for women of ethnic origin since it disrupts the melanocytes and may cause significant permanent scarring.

Thank You

This book was inspired by ethnic women who possess an inner beauty that is hidden by outward scars and feelings of shame and inadequacy. Thank you for teaching me and sharing stories that highlight your truth. Thank you for allowing me to find solutions that address your many complex challenges. Fulfilling this purpose allowed me to sharpen my skills in pursuit of helping you change your narrative. Thank you for allowing me to make a difference in your lives.

I would like to thank all my family and friends, educators, patients and clients, and associates. Because of your support, encouraging words and acts, trust and faith in my abilities, kindness to allow me to learn and grow, I am where I am today.

Bonus

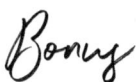

SKIN CARE PRODUCT CHECKLIST

AM

1. Cleanser
2. Toner
3. Moisturizer
4. Sunscreen

PM

1. Cleanser
2. Retinoid
3. Moisturizer

BLEACHING CREAM PRODUCT CHECKLIST

AM

1. Cleanser
2. Bleaching Cream
3. Sunscreen

PM

1. Cleanser
2. Bleaching Cream
3. Retinoid

ANTI-AGING PRODUCT CHECKLIST

AM

1. Cleanser
2. Vitamin C
3. Sunscreen

PM

1. Cleanser
2. Vitamin C
3. Retinoid
4. Moisturizer

ANTI-ACNE PRODUCT CHECKLIST

AM

1. Cleanser
2. Acne Product
3. Sunscreen

PM

1. Cleanser
2. Retinoid
3. Moisturizer

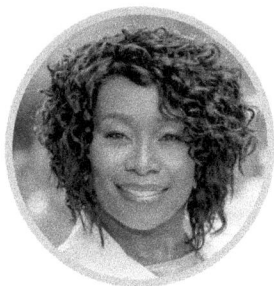

About the Author

Dr. Sonya Campbell Johnson is a national speaker, consultant, creator of the Gorgeous Rx™ System, and board-certified dermatologist who has been in private practice for over twenty years. As the founder and chief medical advisor of DrSonyaJohnson.com, she provides a platform to discuss updated treatments with her clients about their skin concerns. Dr. Johnson is the founder of the virtual dermatology office Derm Elite TeleMed and CEO of Dermatology Associates, PC, a private dermatology practice. Her mission is to help her clients achieve clear and even skin tone with increased confidence through education, lectures, and products.

Dr. Johnson earned her doctor of medicine from St. Louis University and completed her residency at Indiana University. In her spare time, she enjoys running, traveling, reading, cooking, shopping, as well as spending time with her family.

Learn more at SonyaJohnsonMD.com

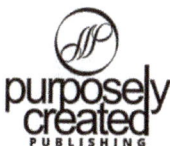

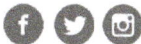